# Pressing RESET for the Remote Worker

original
**strength**

# Öriginal
## strength

*Pressing RESET for The Remote Worker*

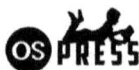

OS PRESS

Published by OS Press, Fuquay-Varina, NC

Contributor: Rob Brinkley Jr, Original Strength Certified PRO - ACE Certified Personal Trainer - ACE Group Fitness Instructor - NASM Performance Enhancement Specialist

ISBN: 978-1-963675-09-2 (Paperback)

As a remote worker, you get to skip the commute, have some flexibility with your schedule, and dress casually from the waist down.

But sometimes, that freedom slowly creeps away. The lines between work and home blur, and you find yourself sitting longer than a marathon runner takes to complete a 26.2-mile run.

> Sitting for extended periods isn't setting your body up to express its best self.

Sitting for extended periods isn't setting your body up to express its best self. It often zaps you of your energy, and further reduces activity throughout your day.

**You can take back the freedom and flexibility of your remote lifestyle!**

Reclaim your health and vitality with Original Strength's RESETs, and do something to help you feel better and move better.

By incorporating these simple yet effective movements, you can regain your energy, boost your productivity, and enjoy the perks of remote work without sacrificing your well-being.

It's time to Press RESET and rediscover the joy of feeling great every day.

In your home office:

If your router has a hiccup, you reset it.

If you can connect to the router but see the message "no internet," it's time to reset your internet connection.

What if your VPN starts slowing down or gets glitchy?

When you call your IT department. What's the first thing they ask? "Did you reset it?" If you disconnect and reconnect the VPN, they'll follow up with, "Did you reset the computer?"

If a device isn't working correctly, you press reset on it.

Your body needs a reset, too.

Pressing RESET on your body can restore and maintain your natural movement patterns and reflexive strength. Modern lifestyles, with their sedentary habits and repetitive motions, cause us to lose the natural, efficient movements we had as children.

Think of your Original Strength as your home office's internet connection.

When you're stuck on dial-up, everything feels sluggish and glitchy, and you get disconnected easily—just like when your body has been sitting too long or stuck in repetitive motions.

But Pressing RESET is like upgrading to DSL—things start moving more smoothly, and you feel more connected. Practice consistently, and it's like upgrading to fiber optic internet: fast, reliable, and effortlessly robust. Like resetting your electronics keeps them running at their best, Pressing RESET helps your body reclaim its natural strength and vitality.

## Ready to rediscover your original strength and live life to the fullest?

# Important Note

Exercise has risks associated with it. Research shows it can lead to being stronger, healthier, and happier. However, it can also lead to injuries or even death. It happens.

You should also know that doing nothing also has risks associated with it. Research shows that being sedentary can lead to sickness, weakness, frailty, depression, and anxiety. It can also make you more injury-prone and hasten your destination towards death. It happens.

Consult your trusted family physician before beginning any exercise program or engaging in any sedentary lifestyle.

# Pressing
# RESET

# The Pressing RESET Method

Original Strength's Pressing RESET Method consists of five developmental movement patterns:

1. **Nasal Belly Breathing**
2. **Head control**
3. **Rolling**
4. **Rocking**
5. **Cross-crawl movements**

(We call them RESETS)

These developmental movement patterns restore ("reset") your central nervous system, stimulate your vestibular system, and enhance the communication and functioning of your Nervous, Vestibular, and Muscular systems.

## Why is this important?

If your nervous or vestibular system isn't functioning optimally, your body will put the brakes on your movement patterns.

Your brain's primary goal is to protect you. It will limit what it doesn't think you are capable of doing.

This protective mechanism prevents you from fully expressing and living your best life.

# Pressing
# RESET

# Breathing (with your belly)

Sitting at your desk for hours, dealing with deadlines, and constantly staring at screens can lead to shallow, chest-based breathing.

This type of breathing keeps your body in a constant state of low-level stress, contributing to fatigue, tension, and decreased productivity.

> **Belly breathing, activates your parasympathetic nervous system.**

Belly breathing, on the other hand, activates your parasympathetic nervous system—the "rest and digest" system—helping you relax, focus, and perform better.

When you engage in belly breathing, you increase oxygen flow to your brain and body, which boosts your energy levels and enhances mental clarity. It's like giving your internal operating system a much-needed software update, ensuring everything runs smoothly and efficiently.

# Why Nose Breathing Matters

Breathing through your nose might seem like a small detail, but it profoundly impacts your body and mind. Unlike mouth breathing, nose breathing filters, warms, and humidifies the air you breathe, preparing it for optimal absorption by your lungs. This simple act helps keep your airways moist and clean, reducing the risk of respiratory issues.

Nose breathing activates the diaphragm more effectively, promoting deep, full breaths that improve oxygen exchange. This increased oxygen supply to the brain enhances cognitive function, sharpens focus, and boosts productivity.

# Try this: Supine Belly Breathing

## BELLY BREATHING THROUGH THE NOSE

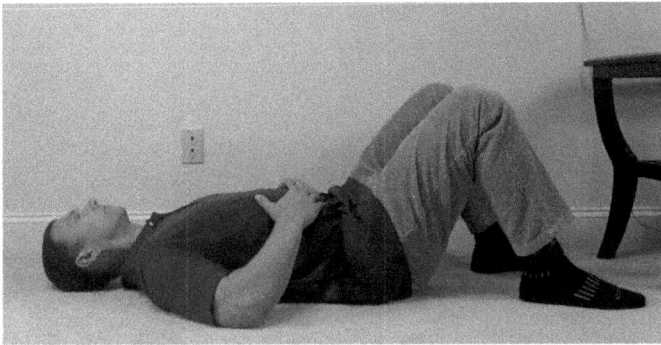

- Place your hands on your belly.
- Put your tongue behind your teeth.
- Inhale through your nose, filling and expanding your belly.

*Your hands should rise and fall with each breath. Bonus points if you visualize expanding your lower ribs out to your sides.*

Set a timer for 5 minutes.

Get comfortable and start practicing.

# Try this: Modified Child's Pose Breathing

## BELLY BREATHING THROUGH THE NOSE

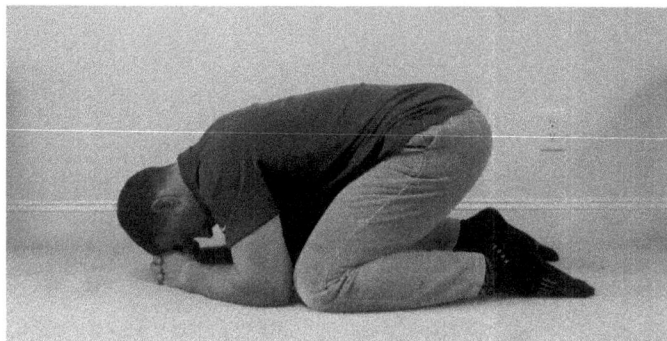

- Bring knees to elbows.
- Rest your head on your fists.
- Put your tongue behind your teeth.
- Inhale through your nose, filling and expanding your belly.

*You can think of your legs as mild resistance to expand/ breathe into.*

Set a timer for 5 minutes.

Get comfortable and start practicing.

# RESET 2

## Head Control

When you were a kid, you had a huge head.

Statistically, it was 33% of your entire body weight.

Learning to move that big lunkhead around was impressive.

Mastering head control back then wasn't just about not falling over and faceplanting. It was about building a strong core. It was about strengthening your vestibular system—the unsung hero of your balance and coordination.

> For remote workers, keeping your vestibular system active is a game-changer.

This system is your body's internal gyroscope, helping you stay balanced and coordinated. Every muscle in your body is in cahoots with this system, making it essential for smooth and efficient movement.

For remote workers, keeping your vestibular system active is a game-changer. The more you move your head, the more you stimulate this system and improve the communication lines between your brain and muscles. Think of it as upgrading your body's software for optimal performance.

*If practicing head movements make you feel dizzy, stop. Practice some deep belly breathing until you no longer feel dizzy. Then try again another time.

Start where you are and do what you can.

# Try this: Supine Head Control

**(HEAD NODS)**

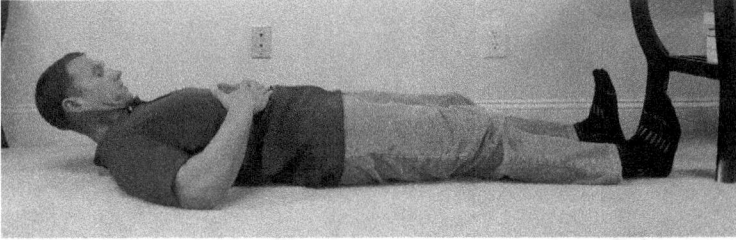

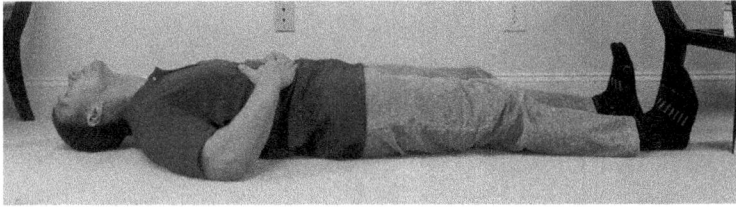

- Place your tongue behind your teeth.
- Keep your mouth closed.
- Move only within your pain-free range of motion.
- Lead with your eyes - tuck your chin and look at your feet.
- Lead with your eyes - try to look above your head.

Set a timer for 1 minute and start practicing.

# Try this: Supine Head Control

**(HEAD ROTATIONS)**

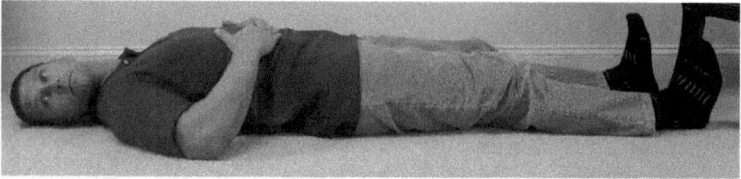

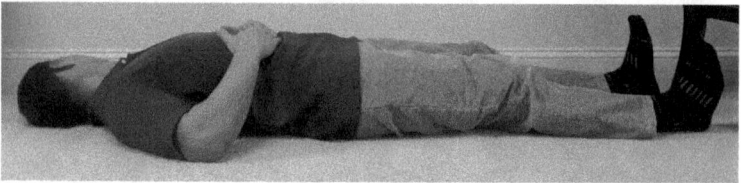

- Place your tongue behind your teeth.
- Keep your mouth closed.
- Move only within your pain-free range of motion.
- Lead with your eyes, then head - look to your left.
- Lead with your eyes, then head - look to your right.

Set a timer for 1 minute and start practicing.

# Try this: Prone TV position Head Control

## (HEAD NODS)

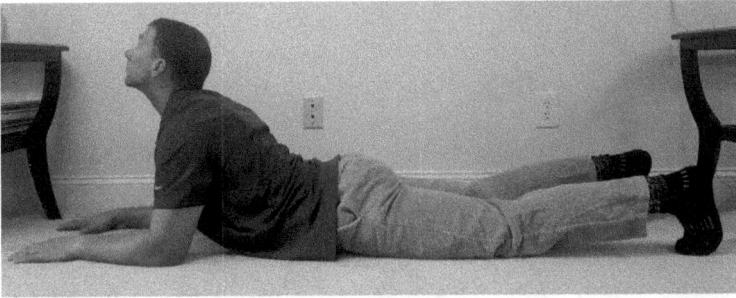

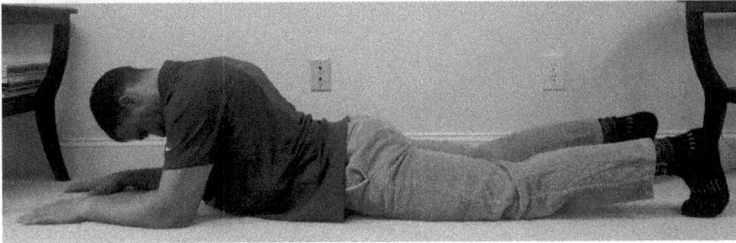

- Place your tongue behind your teeth.
- Keep your mouth closed.
- Move only within your pain-free range of motion.
- Lead with your eyes, then head, and look for the ceiling
- Lead with your eyes, then head, and look for your belly button.

Set a timer for 1 minute and start practicing.

# Try this: Prone TV position Head Control

**(HEAD ROTATIONS)**

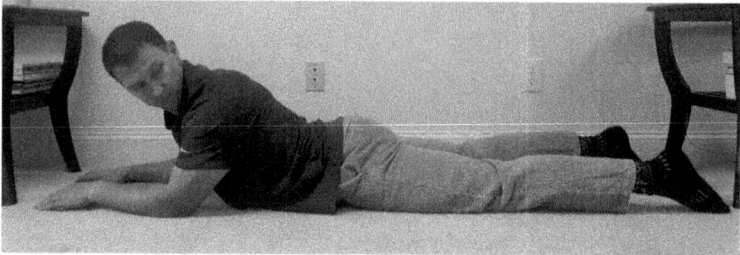

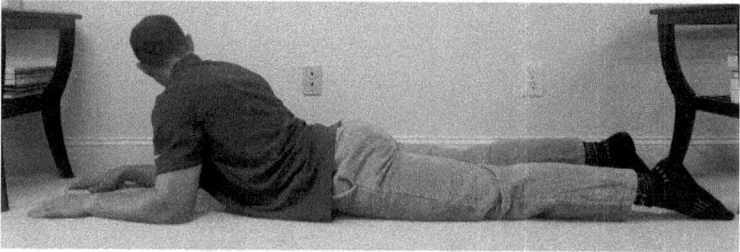

- Place your tongue behind your teeth.
- Keep your mouth closed.
- Move only within your pain-free range of motion.
- Lead with your eyes - look to your left and find your shoes.
- Lead with your eyes - look to your right and find your shoes.

Set a timer for 1 minute and start practicing.

# RESET 3

# Rolling

Rolling is like hitting the refresh button on your body.

It connects your opposite shoulder to your opposite hip, nourishing your spine and stimulating your skin, fascia, and muscles.

It also activates your vestibular system—the key player in your balance and coordination game.

> **Rolling is like hitting the refresh button on your body.**

The following few pages will introduce you to some gentle rolling options. Try them all, see which works best for you, and start practicing.

Set a timer for 1-2 minutes and get rolling.

If rolling makes you dizzy, pause. Then, practice deep belly breathing until you feel steady, and try again.

# Try this: Egg Roll

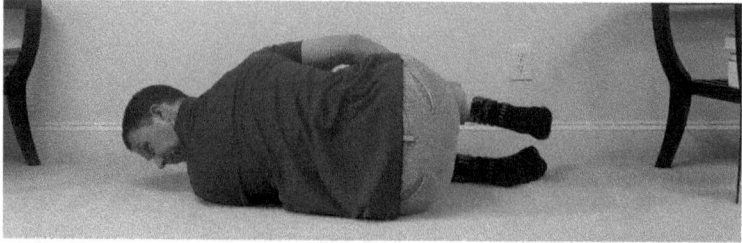

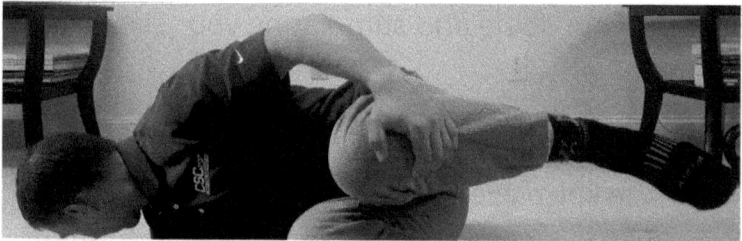

- Lie on your back.
- Hold your knees toward your chest.
- Look with your eyes, then your head, in the direction you want to go and allow your body to roll in that same direction.
- Keep your tongue on the roof of your mouth, breathing via your nose.
- Repeat on the other side, alternating sides with each repetition.

Imagine yourself gently rolling from side to side.

# Try this: Windshield wipers (rotation)

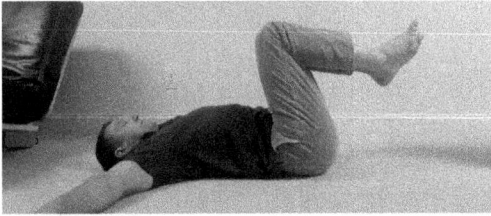

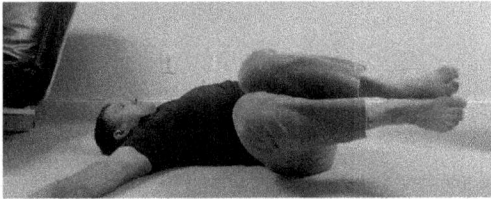

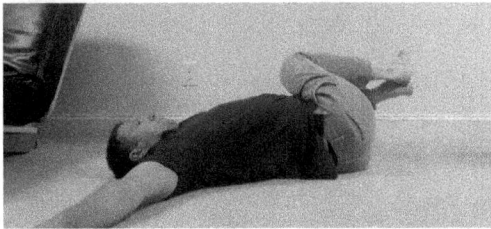

1. Lie down on the floor (or your bed).
2. Arms can reach out straight in a T.
3. Keep your shoulder blades pinned down to the floor.
4. Rotate your legs from side to side.
5. Keep your tongue on the roof of your mouth, breathing via your nose.
6. Alternating sides with each repetition.

# Rocking

Rocking is where you build your strength to crawl and ultimately walk.

## Benefits of Rocking:

- **Activates the Vestibular System:** Rocking stimulates your vestibular system, which is crucial for balance and spatial awareness.

> Tap into the foundational movements of development, enhancing your balance, strength, and posture.

- **Creates Gentle Strength:** Rhythmically rocking gently strengthens your muscles and joints, promoting stability and coordination.

- **Establishes Reflexive Posture:** Rocking helps establish and maintain a reflexive posture, supporting the natural curves of your spine and improving overall posture.

By incorporating rocking into your routine, you tap into the foundational movements of development, enhancing your balance, strength, and posture.

Take a break from your desk and give rocking a try—your body will thank you!

# Try this: Rocking Exercise

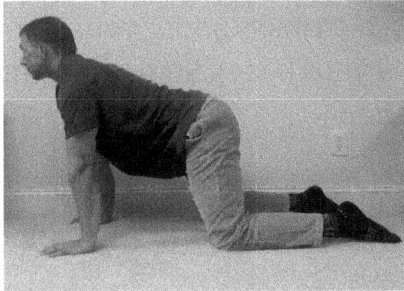

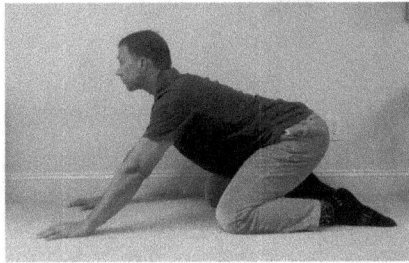

- Gently get down on your hands and knees.

- You can use padding for your knees if necessary.

- Look at the horizon with your mouth closed, breathing in through your nose and filling your belly with your breath.

- Move only within your pain-free range, reaching your hips back toward your feet.

- Rock back to your starting position.

- Repeat the rocking motion.

Practice for 2 minutes

<u>*Additional Rocking tips:*</u>

If your knees are tender, you can put something like a thick mat or couch cushion under your shins (the part of your leg below your knee). Something that gets your kneecap off the floor.

Example:

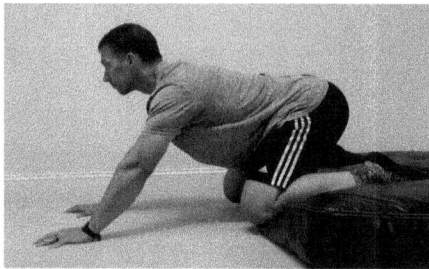

If your wrists are tender, you can use pushup handles.

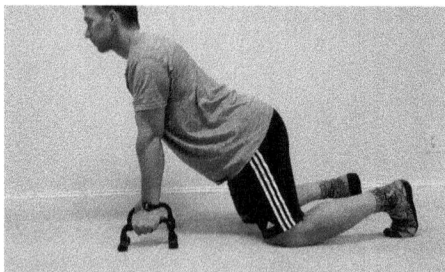

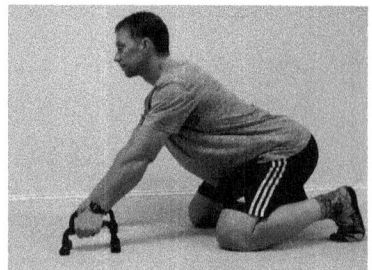

Try a few positions with your feet. First, rock on the tops of your feet, as shown in the original picture.

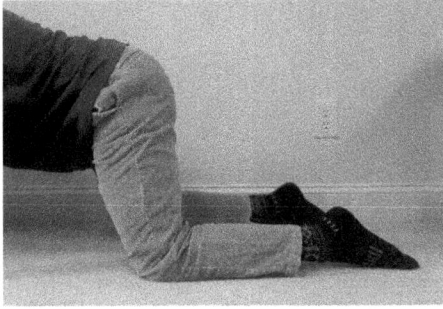

Also, try rocking with your toes tucked under.

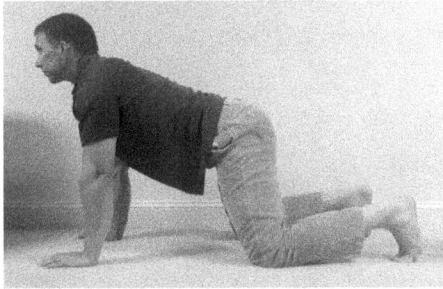

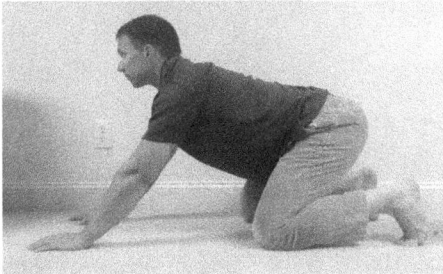

You can also explore different widths (how close your legs are to each other).

Keep your head up.

# Cross Crawl Movements

Cross Crawl Movements pair your opposite limbs (right arm-left leg & left arm-right leg).

The crawling position, in particular, offers extra benefits like strengthening muscles, improving posture, and giving your vestibular system a good workout.

Cross Crawl Movements are like re-wiring your system for peak performance.

This patterning stimulates the brain and boosts connections between the left and right hemispheres, making you smarter and stronger!

> Cross Crawl Movements are like re-wiring your system for peak performance.

And guess what? It's not just about crawling; it works with marching, walking, running, skipping – any activity where you deliberately use all four limbs and pair opposites.

The following pages will give you multiple options to try.

Be curious, play safe, and don't force anything you don't feel comfortable doing.

# Try this: Standing Cross Crawls

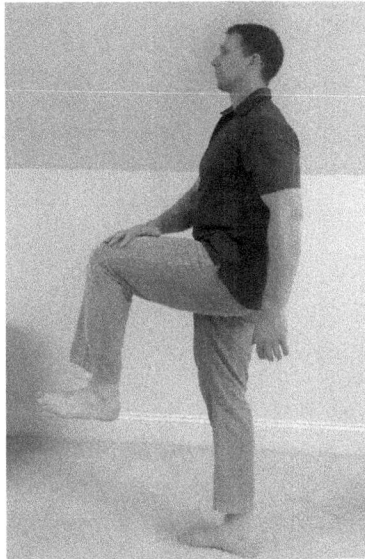

- Lift one leg.
- Touch the opposite hand to that leg (left leg - right hand).
- Switch lifted leg and touched hand.
- Continue practicing and getting comfortable with the movement. You can vary your speeds (deliberately slow, medium pace, and faster) as you go.

Set a timer and practice for 2 minutes.

# Or this: Birddog

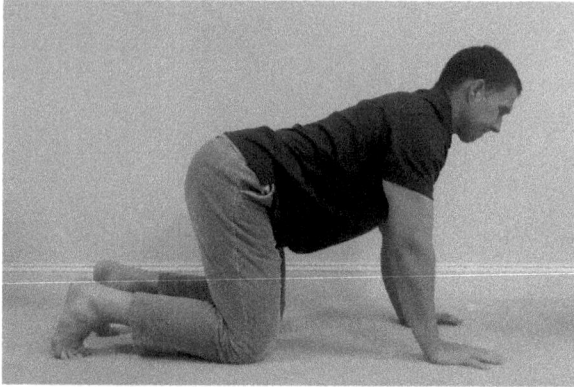

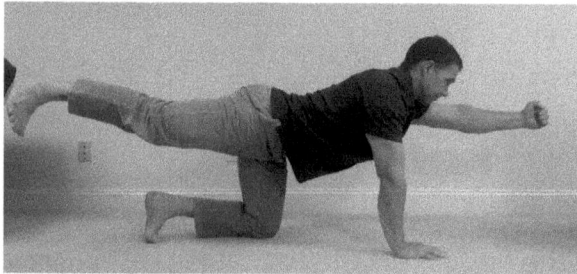

- Start in a 6-point (hands-knees-feet) kneeling stance. Use a knee pad if needed.
- Reach one arm and the opposite leg out in a horizontal line (side view).
- Return those limbs to your start position.
- Lift/reach with the other arm and leg.

Set a timer and practice for 2 minutes.

# Try this: Crawling

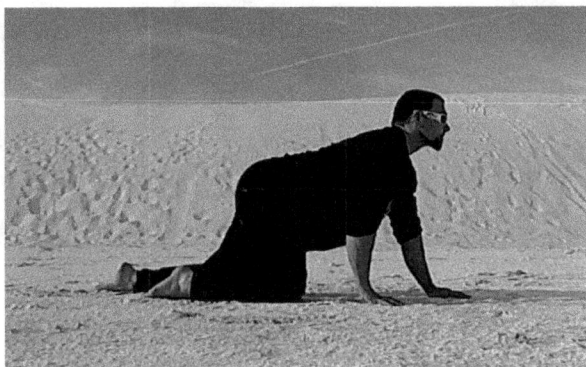

- Start in the same position as rocking.
- Crawl using the opposite arm and leg combo.
- Crawl forward using your right arm and left knee (if the surface allows, drag your feet).
- Repeat left arm and right knee.
- Keep your head up. Don't force it; start where you are.
- If you have a soft surface (mat, carpet, golf course-ish yard), that could be perfect. You could also put on knee pads.
- If your wrists dislike this movement, use the same handles shown in the additional rocking tips.
- Breathe in your nose, with your mouth closed, tongue on the roof of your mouth behind your teeth.

Set a timer and practice for 2 minutes.

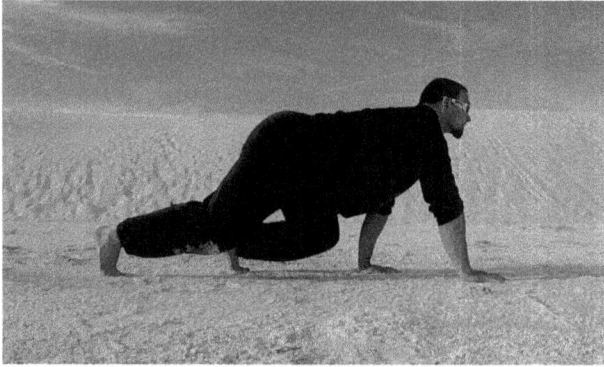

You can also crawl with your knees off the floor.
Your north star would be to keep your hips and back level-ish.

Controlling your breathing will be helpful.
Remember, in your nose with deep belly breaths.

Take breaks as needed.

# Practicing Pressing RESET

The more you practice your RESETS, the more benefits you'll experience.

There's no one right way to practice your RESETS.

> **You can also do a RESET or two at your workstation.**

You can practice them:

- Upon waking in the morning
- For a Mid-day refresh
- After a long day of work
- Before your current exercise routine
- In between sets of your exercise routine
- As a prep for bed

**You can also do a RESET or two at your workstation.**

It can be a quick stress reducer before a big Zoom presentation.

Or you can do a RESET circuit after your daily Zoom meeting.

You can set an alarm to do a RESET every hour.

Whatever works best for you.

The following pages will give you some RESET options you can do at your workstation.

Home Office edition:

# Try this: Seated Belly Breathing

BELLY BREATHING THROUGH THE NOSE

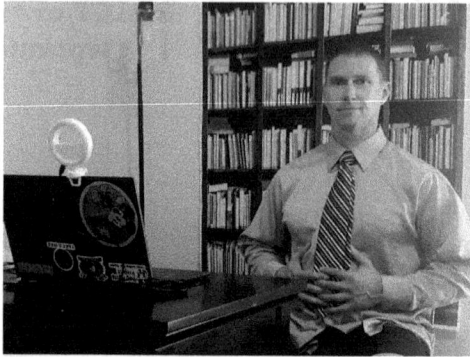

## Seated

- Place your hands on your belly.
- Put your tongue behind your teeth.
- Inhale through your nose, filling and expanding your belly.

*Your aim is for the hands on your belly to move as you breathe.*

Practice for 5 breaths to 5 minutes of breathing.

# Try this: Head Control (Head Nods)

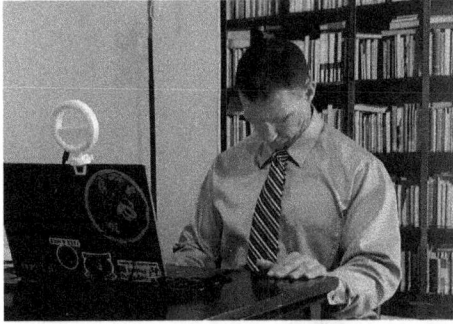

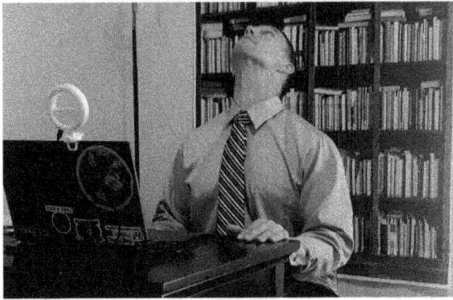

**Seated**

- Place your tongue behind your teeth.
- Keep your mouth closed.
- Move only within your pain-free range of motion.
- Lead with your eyes - look down to the floor.
- Lead with your eyes - try to look above your head.

Practice 10 reps to 1 minute.

# Try this: Head Control (Rotations)

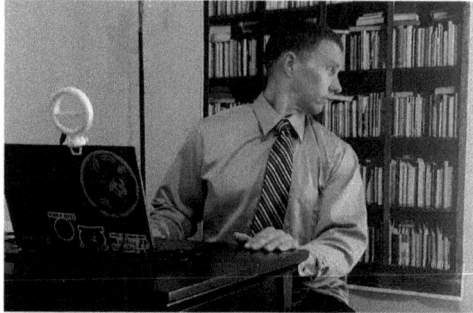

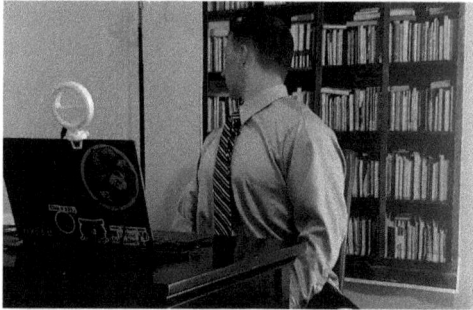

## Seated

- Place your tongue behind your teeth.
- Keep your mouth closed.
- Move only within your pain-free range of motion.
- Lead with your eyes - look to your left and rotate left.
- Lead with your eyes - look to your right, rotate right.

Practice 10 reps to 1 minute.

# Try this: Head Control (Lateral flexion)

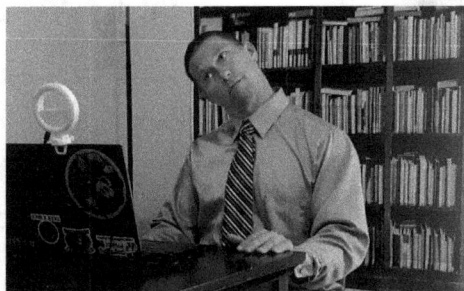

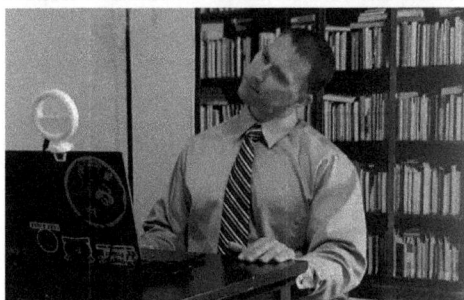

## Seated

- Place your tongue behind your teeth.
- Keep your mouth closed.
- Move only within your pain-free range of motion.
- Fix your eyes on an object in front of you.
- Reach your left ear towards your left shoulder.
- Reach your right ear towards your right shoulder.

Practice 10 reps to 1 minute.

# Try this: Chair Upperbody Roll

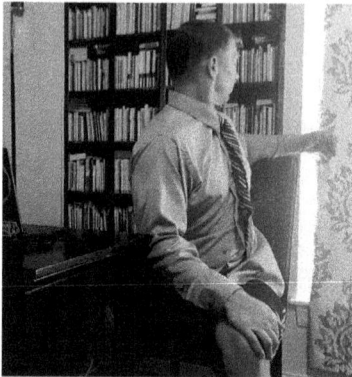

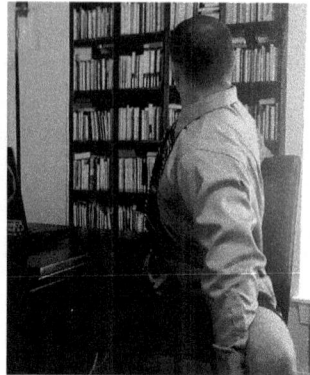

## Seated

- Sit towards the front of a sturdy chair.

- Try to take a wide stance with your legs.

- Look with your eyes, then your head, in the direction you want to go and allow your body to rotate in that same direction.

- Keep your tongue on the roof of your mouth, breathing via your nose.

- Repeat on the other side, alternating sides with each repetition.

Imagine yourself gently rolling from side to side.
Arms can help with rotation. Stay within your pain-free range of motion.

Practice 10 reps to 1 minute.

Pressing RESET for The Remote Worker

# Try this: Standing Lowerbody Roll

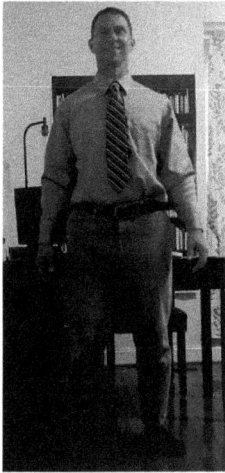

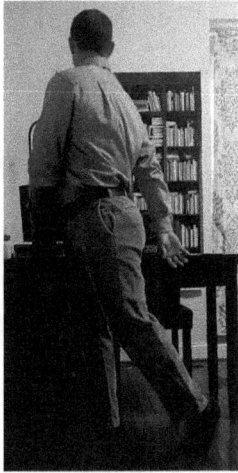

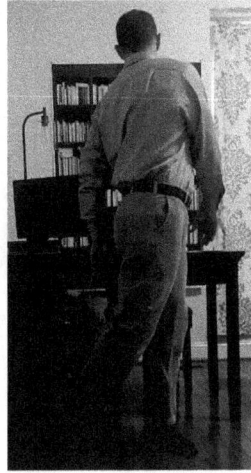

**Standing**

- Stand up tall.
- Look left, with your eyes, then your head
- As you are looking over your left shoulder, at some point, your right foot/hip will want to pivot, let it!
- Repeat on the other side, alternating sides with each repetition.
- Keep your arms loose and free to swing.
- Keep your tongue on the roof of your mouth, breathing via your nose
- Only work within your pain-free range of motion.

Practice 10 reps to 1 minute.

# Try this: Hands elevated Rocking

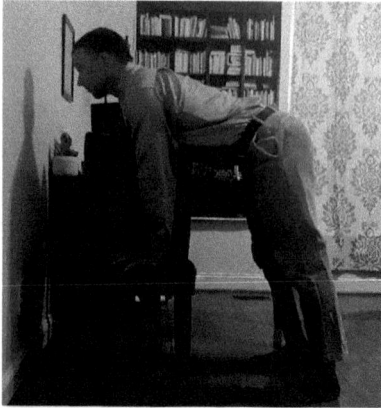

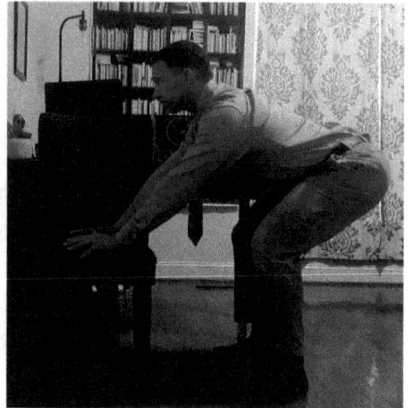

- Place your hands on a sturdy chair or desk.
- Look at the horizon with your mouth closed, breathing in through your nose and filling your belly with your breath.
- Move only within your pain-free range.
- Reach your hips back toward the wall behind you.
- Try to keep the soles of your shoes glued to the floor.
- Rock back to your starting position.
- Repeat the rocking motion.

Practice for 20 reps to 2 minutes

# Try this: Seated Cross Crawls

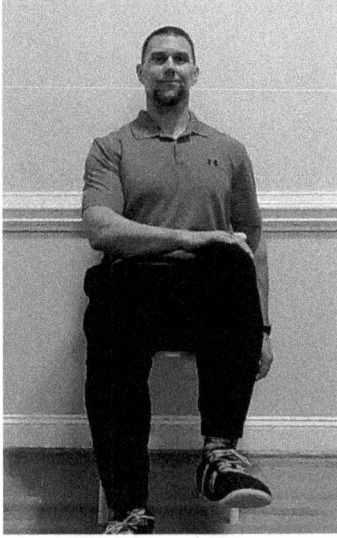

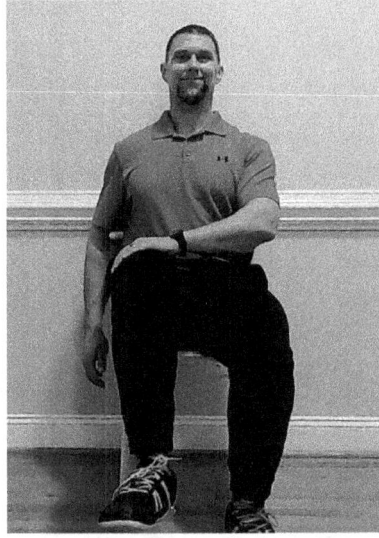

- Lift one leg.
- Touch the opposite hand to that leg (left leg - right hand).
- Switch lifted leg and touching hand.
- Continue practicing and getting comfortable with the movement. You can vary your speeds (deliberately slow, medium pace, and faster) as you go.

Practice for 20 reps to 2 minutes

# Put it all Together:

Practicing all these developmental movement patterns will reestablish healthy communication between your muscular, nervous, and vestibular systems.

This will allow you to move better and feel better about moving!

You don't have to practice all of the included exercises. Try the ones you can. Regularly, pick at least one from each of the 5 developmental movement patterns (RESETS).

Keep it quick, simple, and fun.

Explore the movements. How do they feel?

How do you feel afterward?

*I love the idea of setting a timer every hour or two and practicing a few minutes of resetting your body during your workday!*

Play with the movements every day.

Be creative, have fun, and always work within your pain-free wheelhouse.

# If you want a more structured practice:

Practice 1 to 3 times per day.

- Breathing (with your belly via your nose) - 5 mins
- Head control (head nods) - 1 min
- Head control (rotations) - 1 min
- Rolling - 1-2 mins
- Rocking - 2 mins
- Cross crawl (Marching leg tap) - 2 mins

*Add new (or) reinstate active hobbies that you enjoy!

If you practice for 30 days, how do you think you would feel?

You may notice that you are ready to return to some old hobbies you stopped doing because you weren't feeling as great as you used to.

# Congratulations!

You have completed reading the Pressing RESET for Remote Workers.

By practicing these movements, you are on your way to rediscovering your Original Strength and living life to the fullest.

Keep exploring, stay curious, and enjoy your journey!

# About Our Contributor:

Fitness has been Rob's passion for over 30 years. It all began in a Midwest basement in 1993 with lifting weights, eventually leading to competing in bodybuilding, powerlifting, and even completing five half marathons.

With 16 years of experience as a personal trainer, Rob has earned numerous certifications, reflecting his commitment to continuous learning and professional development. He is a personal trainer at the Original Strength Institute in Fuquay-Varina, North Carolina.

Rob believes in the power of movement and strength training to enhance overall well-being and quality of life. His greatest reward is helping others discover and achieve their full potential.

Connect with Rob: **robertthebrinkley@gmail.com**

# Want to learn more?

This booklet is designed to give you a brief overview of Original Strength's Pressing RESET method. We've crafted this booklet with a singular goal: to empower you to unlock your full potential. The transformative power of the Pressing RESET method can help you feel better, move better, and achieve a level of performance you may not have thought possible. Even if

you only implement a fraction of what's in this booklet; you'll notice significant changes in how your mind and body respond to various situations.

Original Strength Systems (OS) is the leader in nervous system restoration and development of reflexive strength. Our mission is to bring the hope and strength of movement to every body in the world. We provide accredited continuing education courses and books for health, fitness, and education professionals, empowering them to deliver better outcomes to their patients, clients, athletes, and students.

Based on the human developmental sequence, a series of movements that all humans naturally go through as they grow, and the human body's design, OS' Pressing RESET method teaches movements that help RESET an individual's neuromuscular system, allowing them to enjoy improved physical movement and physiological function.

If you want to learn more about Pressing RESET and reclaiming your original strength, https://originalstrength.net is your gateway. There, you'll discover a wealth of resources, from comprehensive books to hundreds of free video tutorials (OS Movement Snax) and a complete directory of our courses and OS Certified Professionals in your vicinity.

We're here to support you every step of the way. If you're ready to enhance your movement system, we encourage you to connect with an OS Certified Professional. They can conduct an Original Strength Screen and Assessment (OSSA), a quick and simple method to identify areas for improvement. With the OSSA, the professional can guide you to the most effective starting point for your journey to restore your Original Strength through the Pressing RESET technique.

Remember, the OS team is always here for you. If you have any questions or need further guidance, please don't hesitate to reach out. We're committed to your journey towards better movement and health.

Please keep us updated on your progress. We want to know how you are doing. Progress@OriginalStrength.net

**Press RESET now and live life better and stronger** because you are awesomely and wonderfully made to accomplish amazing things.

For more information:

# ⏻riginal
## strength

Original Strength Systems, LLC
OriginalStrength.net

PressingRESETfor@Originalstrength.net

"... I am fearfully and wonderfully made..."
Psalm 139:14

www.ingramcontent.com/pod-product-compliance
Lightning Source LLC
Chambersburg PA
CBHW070032030426
42335CB00017B/2393